The Turtle Diet

The slow and steady way to lose weight

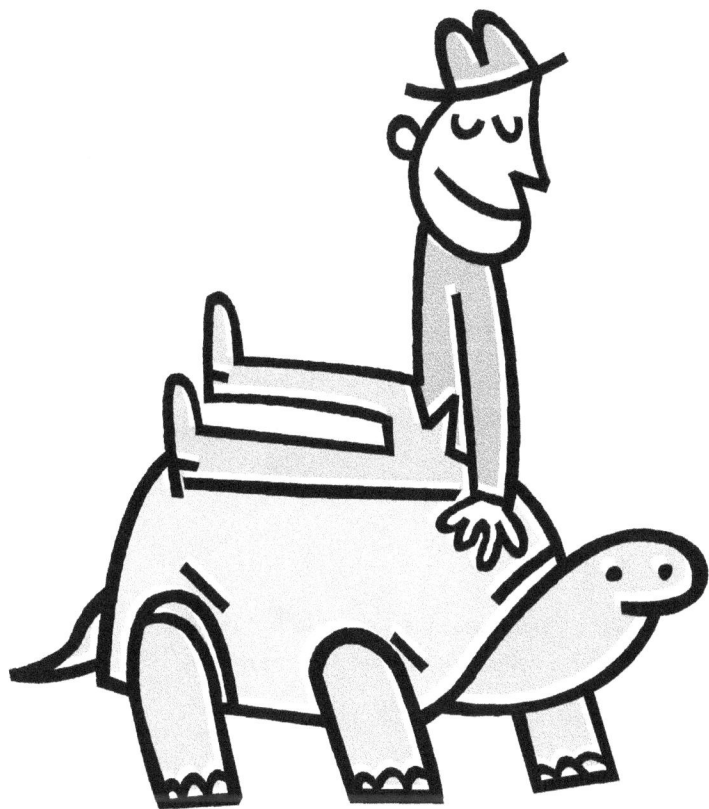

Kevin Carroll

The Turtle Diet is available online.

ISBN: 978-0-9819608-2-1

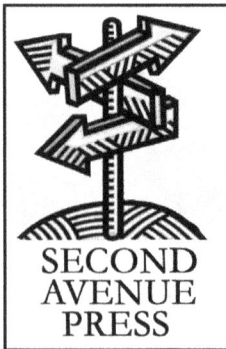

SECOND
AVENUE
PRESS

To Aunt Clare...
The youngest 80-year-old I know

You have to stay in shape.
My grandmother, she
started walking five miles a
day when she was 60.
She's 97 today and we don't
know where the hell she is.

Ellen Degeneres

Foreword

First things first. I'm not a doctor, nutritionist, dietitian or personal trainer. I'm the guy next door who never had much self-discipline when it came to dieting or losing weight.

One day, while pondering how I was going to get rid of the 10 to 15 pounds that I had been carrying around for too many years, it hit me. I realized that I didn't care how much *time* it took me to loose weight, just as long as I lost it. I also figured that if I lost just a little weight over a longer period of time, I wouldn't have to change my eating habits much at all. (I hate

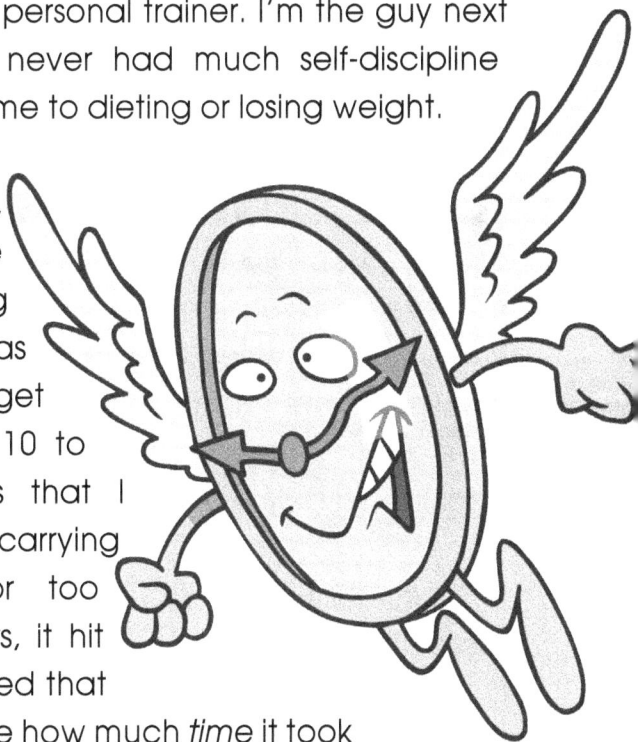

changing habits.) All I'd have to do would be to make ever-so-slight adjustments along the way and *time* would take care of the rest. So that's when I created *The Turtle Diet*. A diet (or better yet, a "mindset" or "lifestyle") that's based on one effortless concept: *Slow and Steady Wins the Race.*

If you're the type of person who wants or needs to lose a lot of weight in a short period of time, then THIS BOOK IS NOT FOR YOU! If, however, you're a patient person *and* you'd like to lose between 10 and 20 pounds (and you hate the idea of making significant changes to your eating habits), then this little book could be just what you're looking for.

I'm sure that there are plenty of diets out there that are fine. It's just that traditional diets don't work for me. I find it too difficult to change my eating habits and to give up the things I love (pizza, candy, chocolate and so on). What I crave is simplicity and ease of use. Thus, *The Turtle Diet* is right for me.

The Turtle Diet is built upon the oldest and simplest concept about weight loss: If you burn more calories than you take in, then you'll lose weight. And, if you're willing to do it *slowly* over an extended period of time, you'll only have to make *minor* changes in your eating habits, you won't get frustrated, and you'll be less likely to put the weight back on. (You didn't gain the extra weight in just two to four weeks, so it doesn't make sense to try and lose it in two to four weeks.)

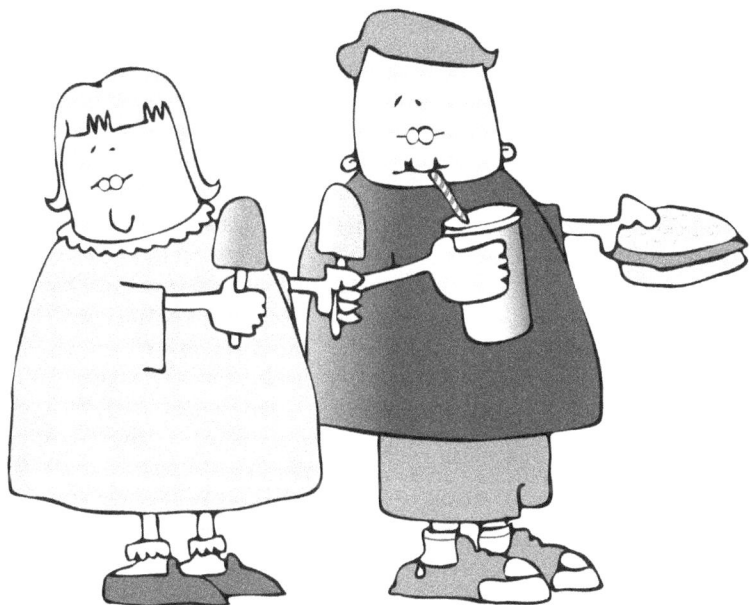

While there are many aspects as to what constitutes a healthy diet, the area I focus on in this book is shaving your caloric intake. Are there other things you should consider besides calories in order to have a well balanced diet? Sure. In fact, I'd encourage you to talk to your doctor about what he or she would recommend. My single-minded goal here is to get you focused on *The Turtle Diet* mindset: slow and steady wins the race.

Perhaps the most important thing you'll take away from this book is this: **100** = **10**. I'll explain what that means in just a bit.

Enjoy the trip.

The other day I saw an ad for The Stump Diet. It said, "Lose nine pounds in one day." That sounded great until I discovered you had to cut your arm off.

Kevin Carroll

The Tortoise and The Hare

There once was a speedy hare who bragged about how fast he could run. Tired of hearing him boast, Slow and Steady, the tortoise, challenged him to a race. All the animals in the forest gathered to watch.

Hare ran down the road for a while and then paused to rest. He looked back at Slow and Steady and cried out, "How do you expect to win this race when you are walking along at your slow, slow pace?"

Hare stretched himself out alongside the road and fell asleep, thinking, "There is plenty of time to relax."

Slow and Steady walked and walked. He never, ever stopped until he came to the finish line.

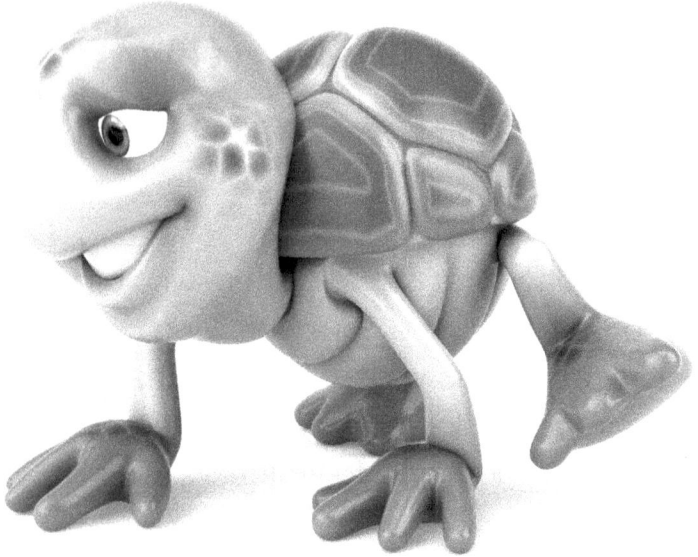

The animals who were watching cheered so loudly for Tortoise, they woke up Hare.
Hare stretched and yawned and began to run again, but it was too late. Tortoise was over the line.

After that, Hare always reminded himself, "Don't brag about your lightning pace, for Slow and Steady won the race!"

Aesop's Fables

The 10 Principles of The Turtle Diet

1. It's All in the Numbers

In order to lose weight you need to burn off more calories than you consume. We all agree, right?

Let's go through the math. There are 3,500 calories in one pound of body fat (give or take a hundred calories). Therefore, if you burn off 3,500 calories more than you consume, you will lose one pound. This, of course, assumes that your weight is stable. (In other words, if you're currently consuming 500 calories a day more than you need just to keep even, and you cut back 100 calories per day, you're still consuming 400 calories more than you need and in less than ten days you'll gain an extra pound!)

Now here's the big news: Over the course of a year, in order to lose ten pounds, you only need (on average) to consume 100 fewer calories per day than you would normally consume. (Again, this assumes you're not consuming too many calories to begin with.)

$$100 = 10$$

So if there's only one thing you remember from *The Turtle Diet*, it should be that 100 calories/day = 10 pounds/year. I believe that if more people realized this fact, we'd all be able to better manage our weight.

Another way to look at it is that the average American male consumes about 2,500 calories per day and the average American female about 2,000 per day. 100 calories equates

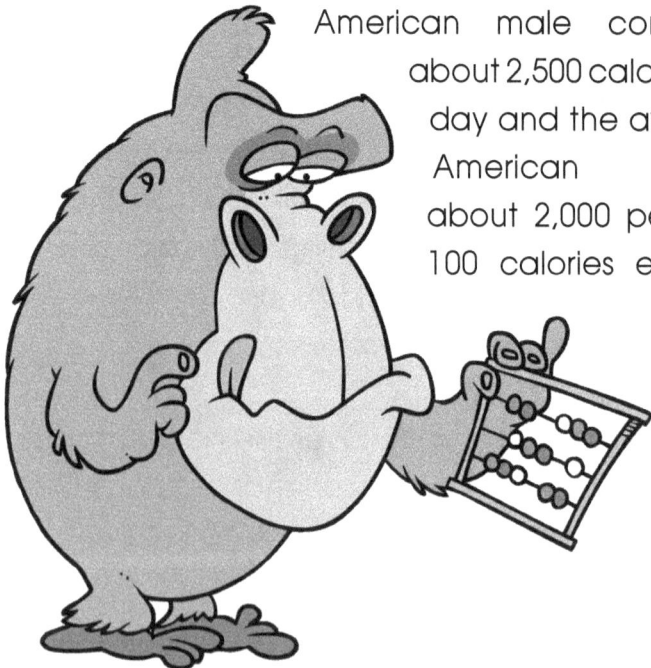

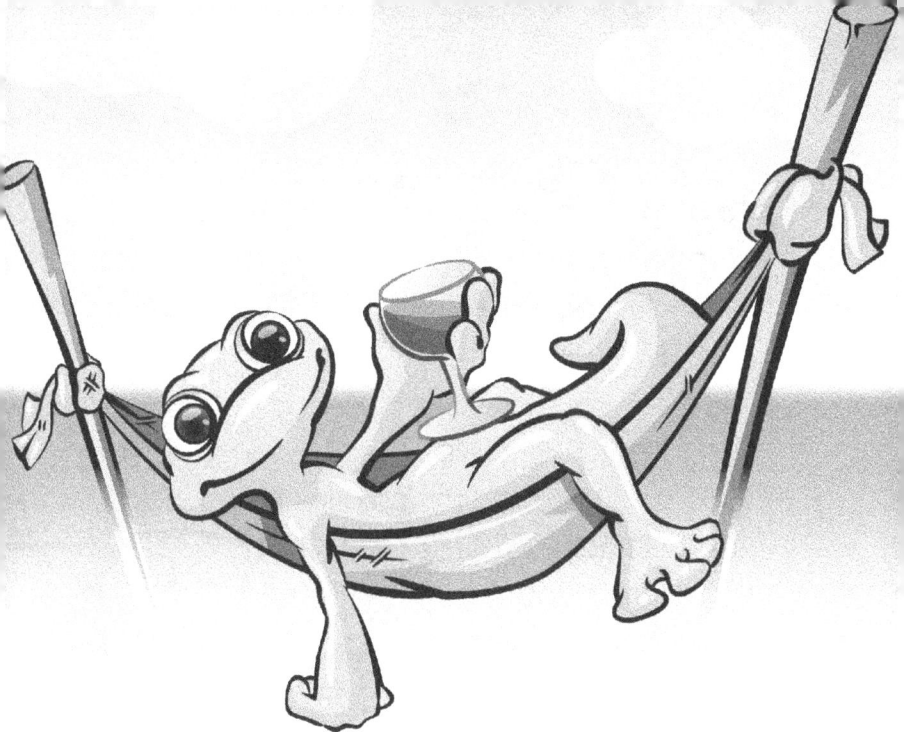

to less than 5% of the average American's daily intake! As they say: "That ain't nothin'."

When you break it down as I have, you start to see that all you have to do is make a *very slight* adjustment in your daily diet (or exercise routine) and you'll lose a noticeable amount of weight *over time*. Remember, *The Turtle Diet* is all about having patience.

Some days you might burn off more than you consume and other days you might consume more than you burn off. No problem. The goal is to burn off more than you consume *over an extended period of time*. Fluctuations are fine and to be expected. YOU MUST HAVE A LONGTERM VIEW.

If you flip to Principle 9, you'll see a list of foods and how many calories each have. And in Principle 10, I've given you a sampling of various exercises and how many calories they burn off. I believe you'll be happily surprised to see that between diet and exercise, all you have to do is make *minor* changes in order to hit your target. If you wanted to be more aggressive and lose 15 pounds a year, then you'd have to consume 150 fewer calories everyday. (200 calories a day equates to 20 pounds and year, 300 calories a day equates to 30

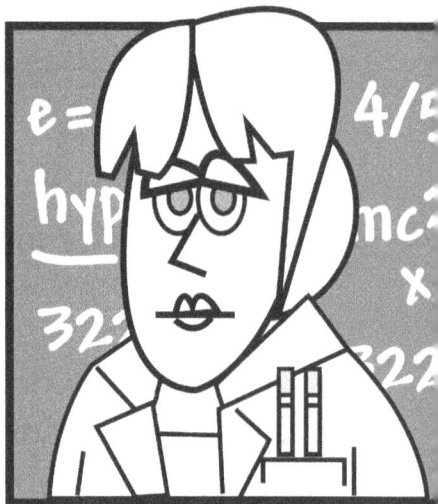

pounds and so on.)

Besides being easy to achieve, the other reason I like 100 = 10 is because it's easy to remember. There's no counting points or weighing food or anything too detailed. Simplicity and common sense are the hallmarks of this diet. All you need to do is get in the habit of glancing at the calories on food and beverage labels. If you consume 100 fewer calories per day (or burn off 100 more calories per day) you'll lose 10 pounds a year or close to a pound a month. An Oreo cookie, for example, has 55 calories and I usually eat four at dessert. If I cut back to two, that will add up to 11.47 lbs. per year! Unbelievable.

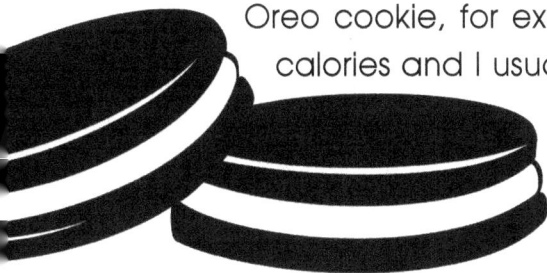

One last thing. I bet that when you try *The Turtle Diet*, you'll find it relatively easy to trim back 100 calories a day and you'll probably be able to cut out more than that with little difficulty. That means you'll likely lose more than you expect and then you'll feel even better because you're ahead of your pace. That will give you encouragement to keep plugging along.

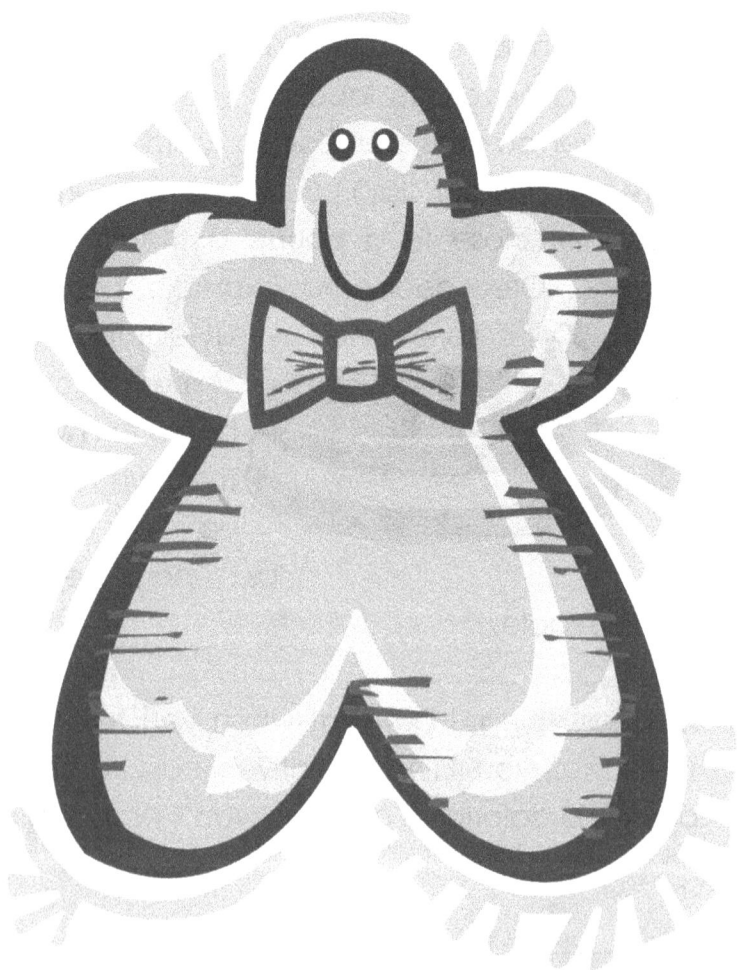

As a point of reference, you can loose 10 to 13 pounds a year if, on a daily basis, you cut back on any ONE of the following:

- Apple Juice, 8 oz. = 120 calories
- Butter, 1 tbsp. = 102 calories
- Mayonnaise, 1 tbsp. = 103 calories
- Olive Oil, 1 tbsp. = 120 calories
- Soda, 10 oz. = 130 calories
- Vodka, 2 oz (80 proof) = 128 calories
- Wine, 6 oz. = 135 calories
- Brownie, 1 oz. = 115 calories
- Apple Pie, 2 oz. = 134 calories
- Chocolate Ice Cream, 3.5 oz. = 125 calories
- Chocolate Chip Cookies, 1 oz. = 136 calories

Note: In order to get a list of every conceivable food, along with its calorie content, do an online search for "Calorie Chart". Also, if you want to determine what your daily caloric intake should be (to simply maintain your weight) do an online search for "Calorie Calculator".

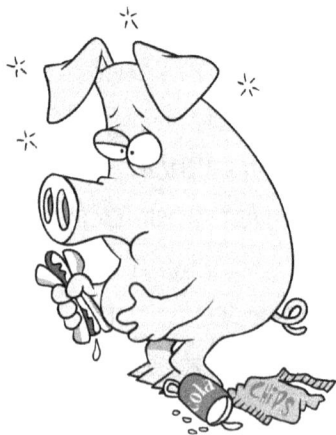

Part of the secret of success in life is to eat what you like and let the food fight it out inside.

Mark Twain

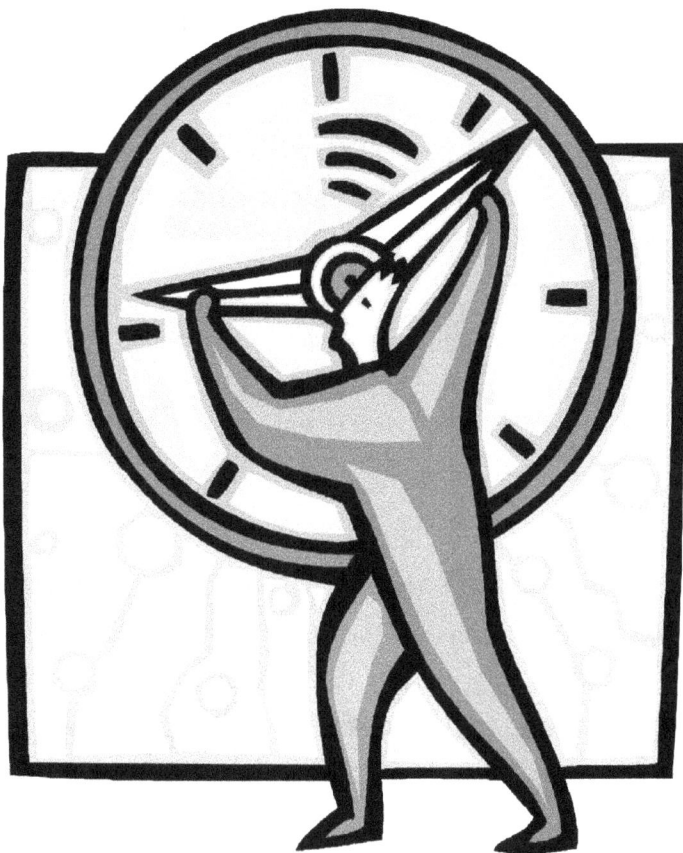

2. Time is Your Best Friend

Let's get right to it. *Patience* is the key to your success on *The Turtle Diet*. As I said in the foreword, if you want a quick fix, this book is not the answer. If, however, you don't need to lose those extra pounds immediately *and* you'd like to stand a better chance of keeping the weight off, then you've come to the perfect place. What this diet hinges on is the idea of making *small* adjustments over a *long* period of time.

Imagine a giant tanker (no, I'm not suggesting you're a giant tanker) heading across the Atlantic from Portugal to Boston. If the captain were to make a *minor* course adjustment early on, then over the course of the trip that tanker would end up in Philadelphia, a significant distance away from Boston. *The Turtle Diet* is based upon the same concept.

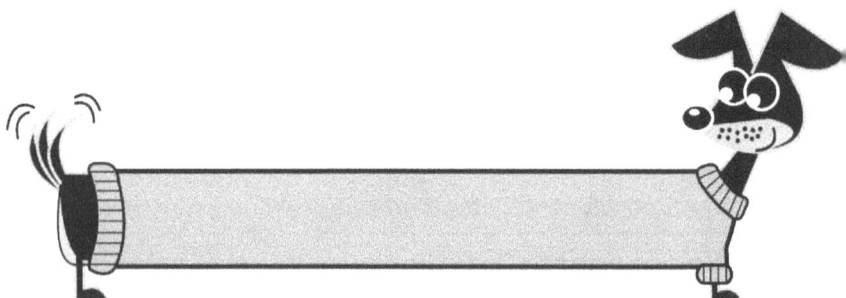

The good news is that when you allow enough time, you won't feel like you're on a diet. In fact, maybe we shouldn't even call this a diet. Maybe the book should be called *The Turtle Attitude* because it should never feel as though you're sacrificing. I'm not into suffering.

So how much time am I talking about? Well it's up to you, but I'm recommending a *minimum* of six months and more like a year to 18 months. Now that may seem like a long period, but, as they say, time flies.

One last thought. If the tortoise and hare were in a 100 yard dash, odds are that the tortoise would lose. Like many of us, the

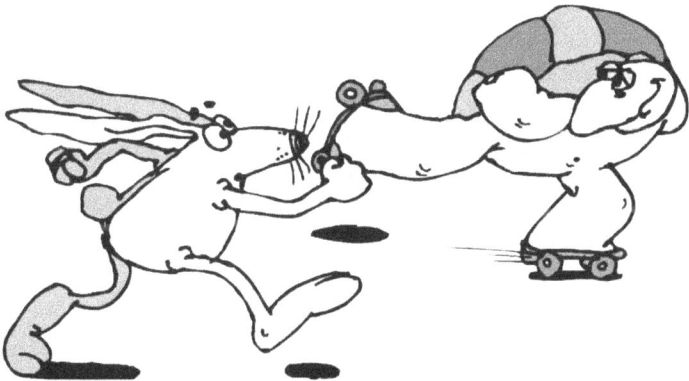

tortoise wasn't built for speed. But over time, little by little, he was able to reach his goal.

So let me repeat myself once again, the essence of *The Turtle Diet* is to make very *small* changes over a *long* period of time vs. making significant changes over a short period of time. Got it?

I've been on a diet for two weeks and all I've lost is two weeks.

Totie Fields

3. No Pain.
No Problem.

Remember when people use to say, "No pain. No gain." That never quite worked for me. I've always believed in finding easier, simpler ways to get things done. Why make things more difficult than they already are?

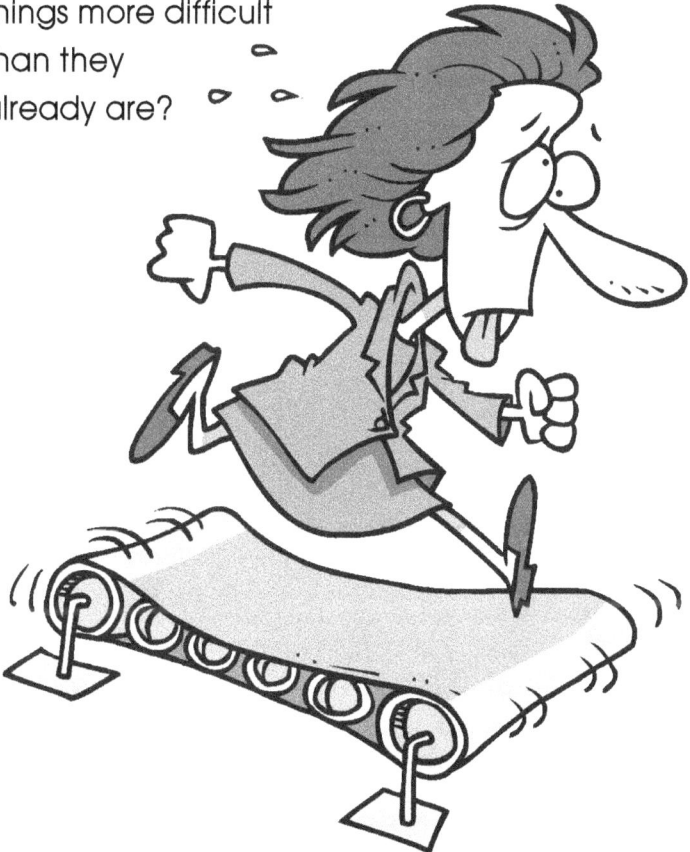

You'll be happy to know that *The Turtle Diet* is based on the principal of **No pain. No problem.** By that I mean that if you ever feel as though *The Turtle Diet* is hard, then you're doing something wrong! This is the most forgiving diet in the world. You can eat whatever you want, whenever you want. (You just can't do it all the time!) The way I figure it, if someone is having a difficult time changing their eating habits and if they're getting totally bummed out when they fall off a diet, then there must be a better way. And there is. By letting *time* help carry the load (so to speak) this diet becomes effortless.

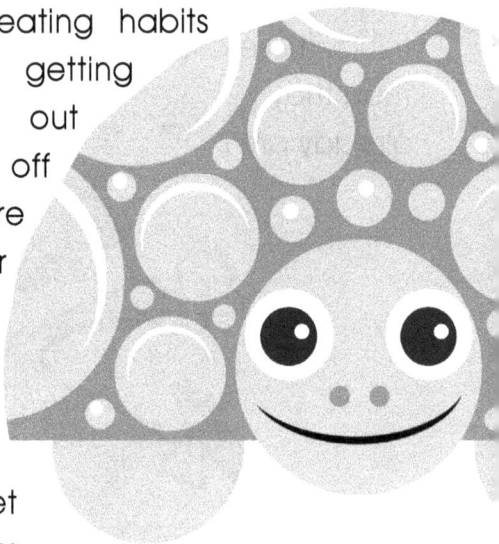

The other day I was out on a bike ride and came across a huge hill. Now normally I'd try to bike up it as fast as I could. This time, however, I changed my approach and decided I'd take it *very* slowly and zigzag my way up the hill so that way the incline wouldn't be too steep. And you know what? It was *so* much easier. Did it take longer to get up the hill? Absolutely. But I made it up without killing myself. The same notion applies to *The Turtle Diet*. Rather than trying to lose the weight as quickly as you can, this diet is all about losing the weight slowly. And that's how you'll be successful.

> *I feel about airplanes the way I feel about diets. It seems to me they are wonderful things for other people to go on.*

Jean Kerr

4. It's Impossible to Fall Off

One of the reasons many diets don't work is because when people fall off them (which they often do), they get discouraged and give up. *The Turtle Diet* is a very tolerant diet and allows you to continue to live your life the way you're used to living it.

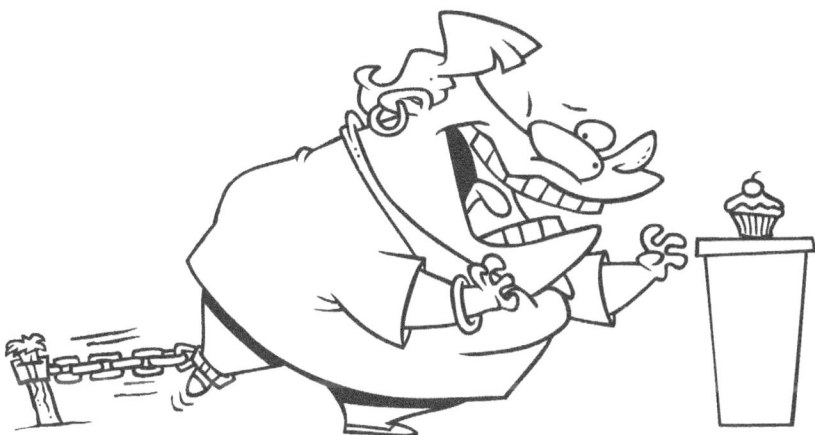

One of the best things about *The Turtle Diet* is that it's impossible to fall off of it because there's nothing to fall off of. If you're trying to cut back on dessert for example, it's perfectly all right to keep having some. All you're trying to do is cut back a little bit - 100 calories a day to be exact. If you have a few days in a row where you haven't cut back on the sweets, that's of little concern. You can cut back on the calories some other place, or you can burn off the calories by getting some exercise. (A 20-minute walk at 4 mph burns off 115 calories.)

Before writing this book, I told a friend about the philosophy of *The Turtle Diet.* She was all excited to try it and told me that she'd

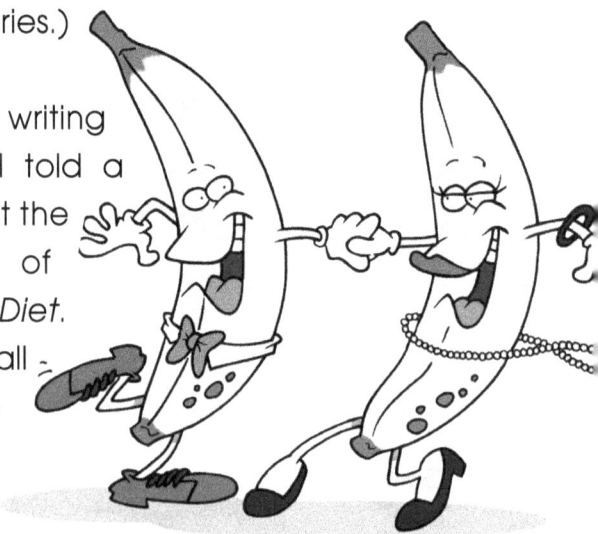

be forever in my debt if I could help her lose weight. A few days later she told me she was so upset because she had binged the night before and fell off the diet. "What do you mean you fell off it? There's nothing to fall off of," I said. Sure, you have good days and bad days, but you can't fall off it. No matter what you eat, if you're still committed to losing the extra weight over the long-term, then you're still on *The Turtle Diet*.

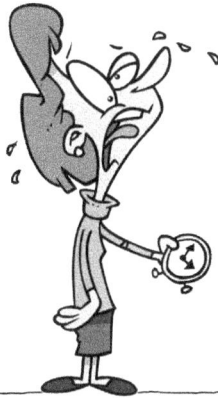

When I started on *The Turtle Diet*, I did great for the first two months. I had lost four pounds over that period of time. Way ahead of my goal of a pound a month. By the end of the third month, however, I had put two pounds back on. I was down on myself and figured that the diet was useless. Then it dawned on me that this diet is all about losing the weight over the long haul. Two months down, one month up, who cares? I was still netting out lower than when I had started, so I was in good shape.

When you find yourself gorging on a bunch of Dunkin' Munchkins, don't worry about it.

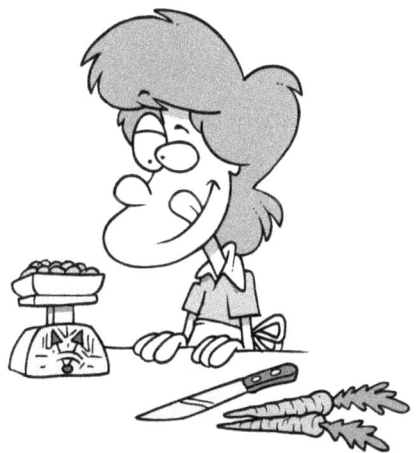

Health food
makes me sick.

Calvin Trillin

5. Know Where You're Going

Any book I've ever read about setting goals always tells you to write your goals down and give yourself a timeframe for accomplishing them. And guess what? Same goes for *The Turtle Diet*. There's something mighty powerful about knowing the specific weight level you want to hit and tracking how you're coming along. It makes the vague concept of losing weight much more tangible.

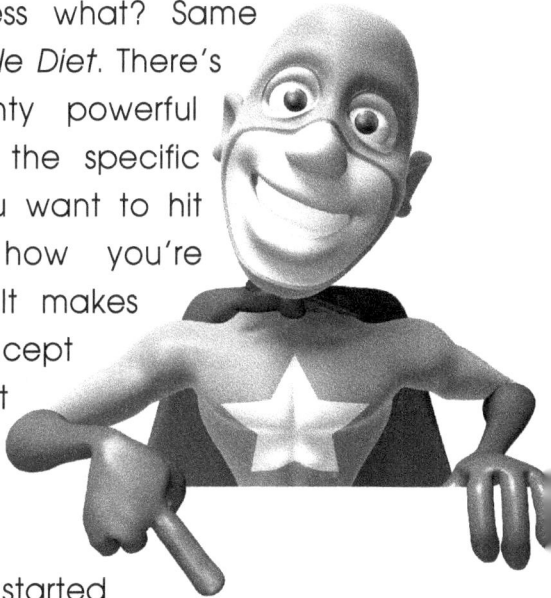

In my case, I started out at 182 pounds and set a goal to lose 17 pounds over 17 months which would get me down to 165 pounds. Knowing my specific target weight gave me something concrete to shoot for.

Would you ever jump in the car with your family and announce, "We're going on vacation!" and have no idea where you were going? Probably not. Same goes for your diet. When you have a goal weight, you have something specific and measurable to shoot for.

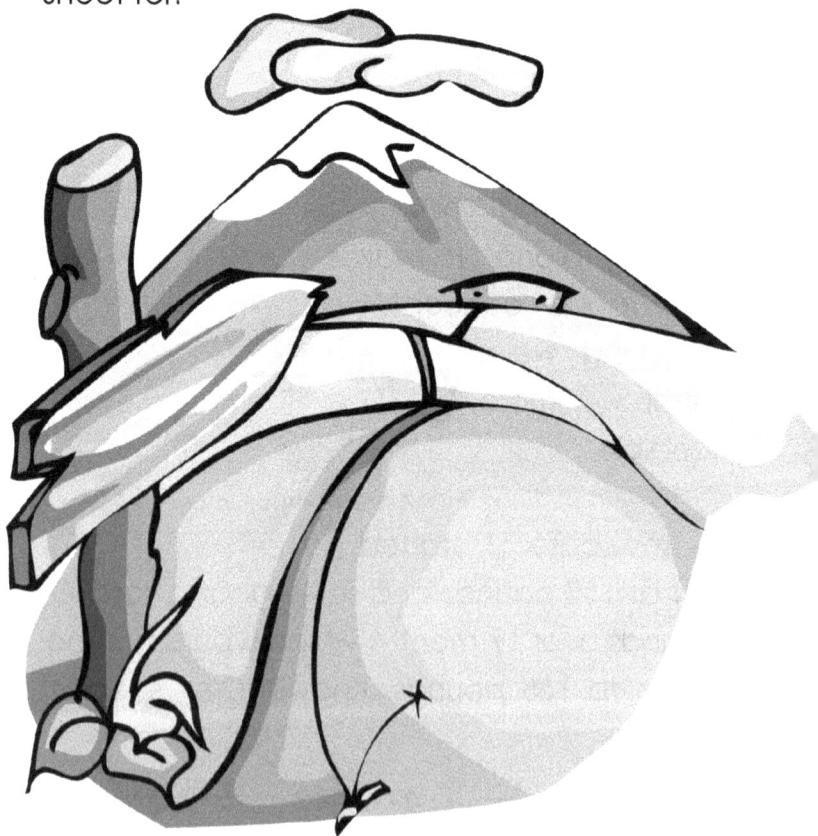

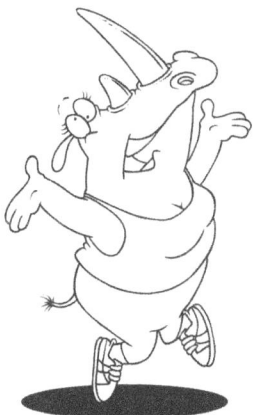

Reminds me of my safari in Africa. Somebody forgot the corkscrew and for several days we had to live on nothing but food and water.

W. C. Fields

6. Don't Weigh Yourself Daily!

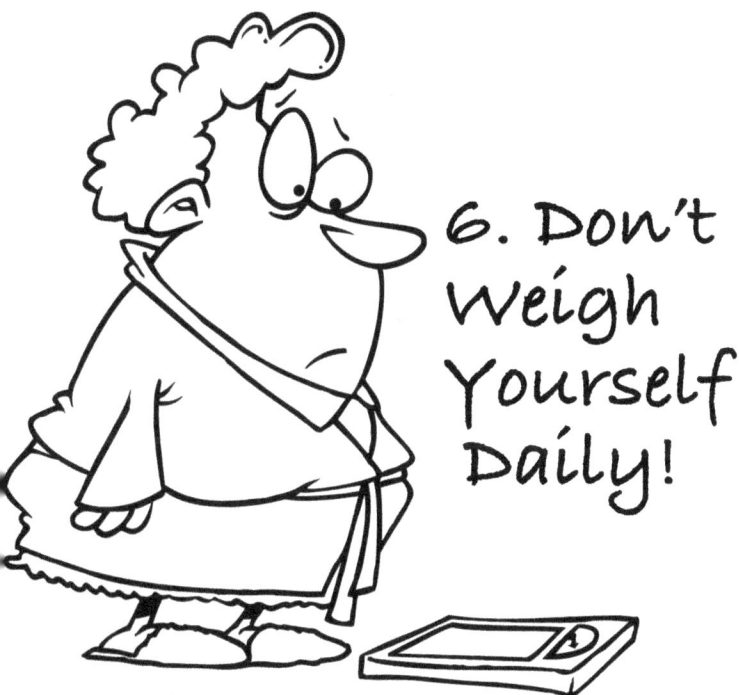

Once you start *The Turtle Diet*, do not weigh yourself every day or even every few days. Fight the urge and weigh yourself once or twice a month. If you weigh yourself more frequently, you'll be too conscious of your weight fluctuations and you'll risk getting down on yourself if your weight goes up. *The Turtle Diet* is intended to be a no hassle diet. Stop torturing yourself with the scale. Allow time to work its magic.

You can pick whatever day of the month you want to weigh yourself. I picked the first of the month because it was easy to remember.

Less is more.

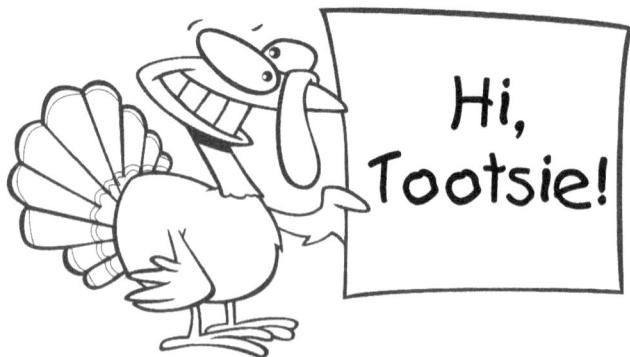

You are what you eat,
so avoid nuts.

Anonymous

7. Chart Your Progress

Just as setting a goal weight is critical (Principle # 5) so, too, is charting your progress. Charting will help make your journey tangible.

In order to get you started, take 5 minutes right now and draw a simple graph for yourself on an 8 1/2 x 11 inch piece of paper.Take a look at the one you see on the next page and create your own version tailored to fit your needs. As you look at the page horizontally, on the left side you'll put your weight. Your current weight will be at the top of the vertical line and your goal weight will be at the bottom of the line. Now along the bottom of the page, draw a horizontal line. The current month will be on the far left side and the target end date will be on the far right side. Finally, draw a straight line from your current weight today (top left of the page) down to your target weight and target end date (lower right side of the page). That's

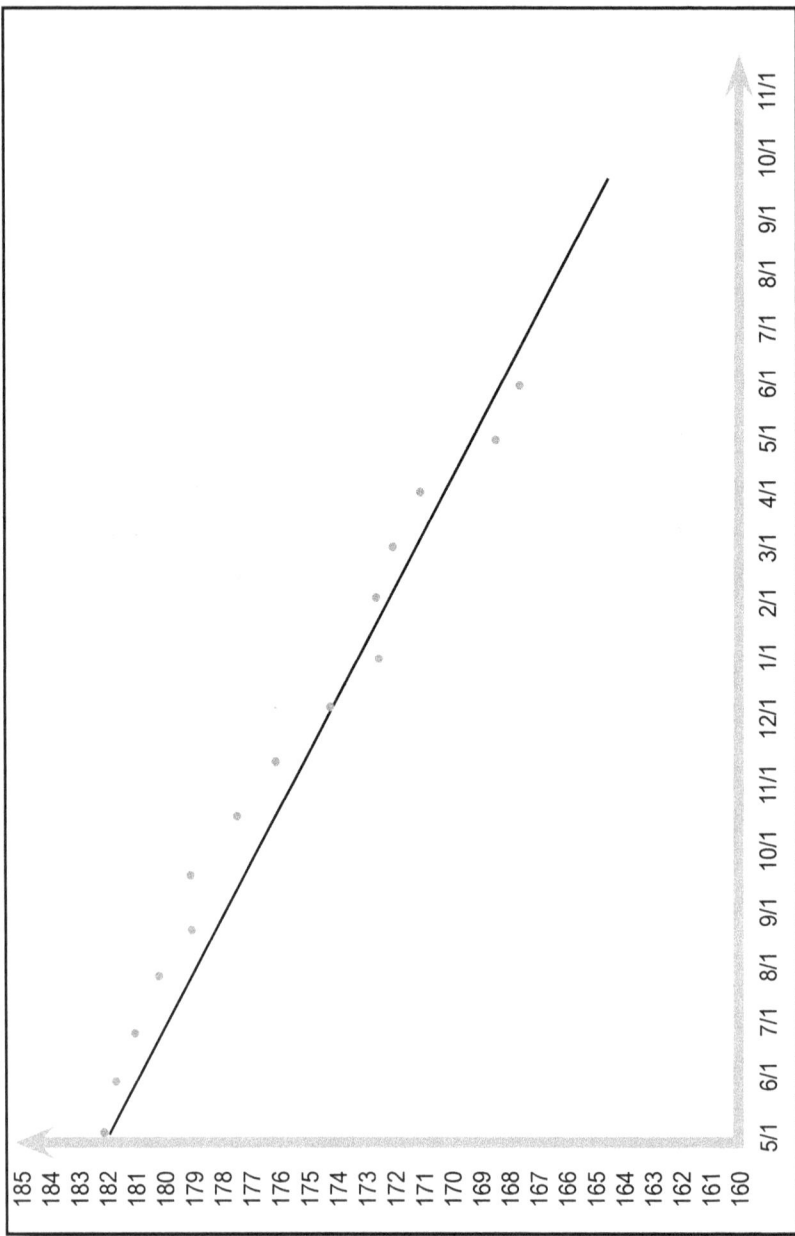

Figure 1

all you need to do. Now you have a visual picture of where you are and where you're trying to get to.

On the first of every month, weigh yourself and mark your weight on the chart drawing a line from your weight the previous month to your weight in the current month. This simple graph worked wonders for me.

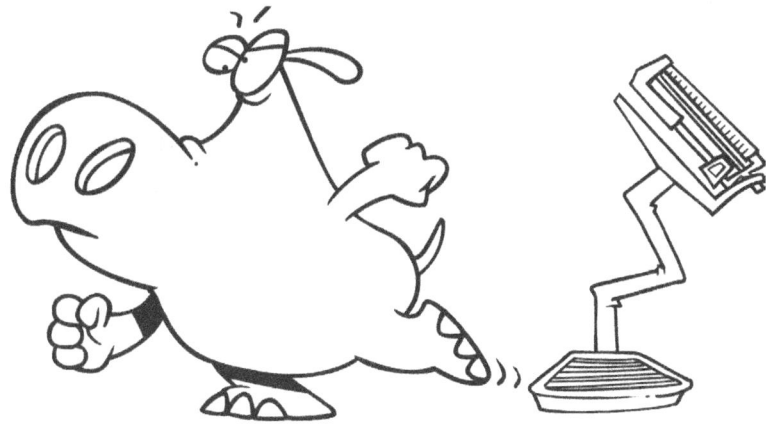

I suggest that you tape your chart to your wall or to some place where you'll be able to see it every day. By keeping your chart visible you'll be able to keep your goal (and your progress) top of mind. Then, on the first of every month, after you weigh yourself, note your weight on the chart. This simple method of charting will help you achieve your goal.

Although the odds are high that your weight will go down every month, there may be some months where you go up a little bit. THIS IS NOT A PROBLEM. Just stick with making the little adjustments and you'll be back on track. If you're like me, you'll meander your way down the chart.

If you want a way to track your progress online, go to: www.EverydayHealth.com and click on the button for "My Calorie Counter"

I come from a family where gravy is considered a beverage.

Erma Bombeck

8. Munch Munch

When it comes right down to the eating part, there are some simple guidelines you'll want to keep in mind. Notice I didn't call them rules. On *The Turtle Diet*, there are no rules.

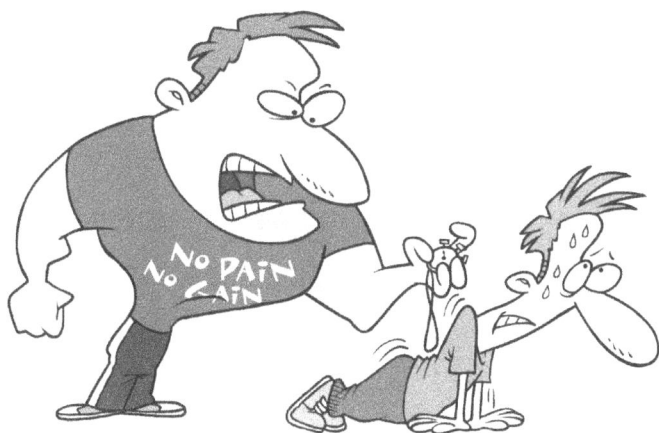

There are guidelines, suggestions, ideas or what have you, but there are no rules. Rules can sometimes be problematic. Especially when you're on a diet, because when you break the rules you can feel dejected and then, before you know it, you give up. Find one or two guidelines that you believe will work well for you and give them a shot. If they help you, then great. However, if they frustrate or annoy you, then drop them and try a different approach. Or make up one of your own. If you feel like you're making a big sacrifice on this diet, then you're doing something wrong.

The suggestions I've shown below are the ones that I like because they're easy and they work for me. Some days I do them and some days I don't, but at least I'm doing *something* and that's what counts. You have to figure out what works best *for you*. For example, a friend of mine is into veggie shakes so she finds it easy to work her concoctions into her daily routine and she's seeing results. Veggie shakes are *her* thing and that's why it's working for *her*. If I had to down a veggie shake, I'd gag. So guess what? Veggie shakes are not one of my guidelines.

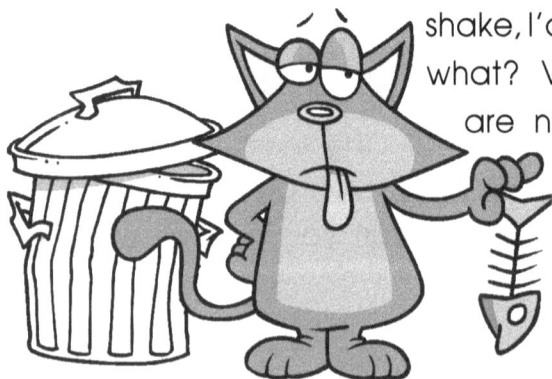

Here's an important consideration: What adjustment can you make to your diet that is going to be easy for *you* to do? If you can't come up with any, do a quick search on the internet and you'll find dozens of ideas.

As I've said before, habits are very difficult to change. If you try to change too many habits at once, you won't change any of them. If you try something new and you can't stick with it, then try something else. The only thing you have to do is make a minuscule improvement over what you're currently doing. Time takes care of the rest.

Ice Cream

Here are some suggestions to get you started. As you'll see, there's nothing revolutionary here. And that's a good thing. These are basic, common sense approaches that countless dietitians and nutritionist would support. Pick a couple that you think you can do and give them a shot. The ones I've listed below are the ones that I find are pretty easy to do.

One last thing. I'm a big believer in the *Post-it Note Theory* of behavior modification. Whatever new behavior you're trying to adopt, write it on three different Post-its and place them strategically around your environs. On your fridge. On your dashboard. On your m o t h e r - i n - l a w ' s forehead. You decide. But place them where you can easily spot them. They'll provide you with gentle reminders

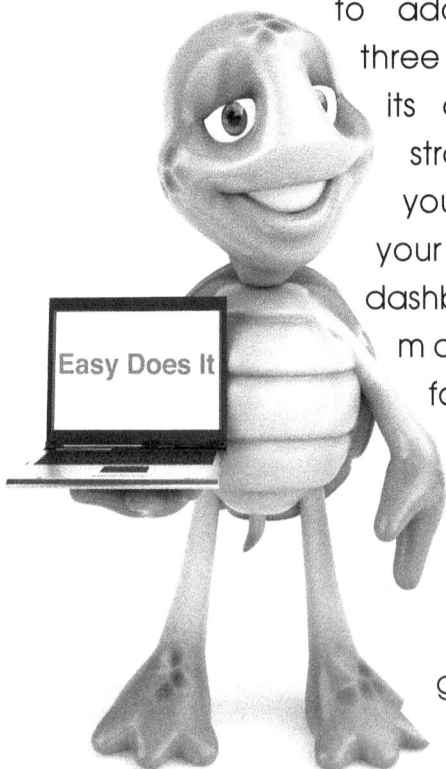

Easy Does It

throughout the day. Humans need to be constantly reminded of the new behavior if they have any real hope of breaking the old behavior.

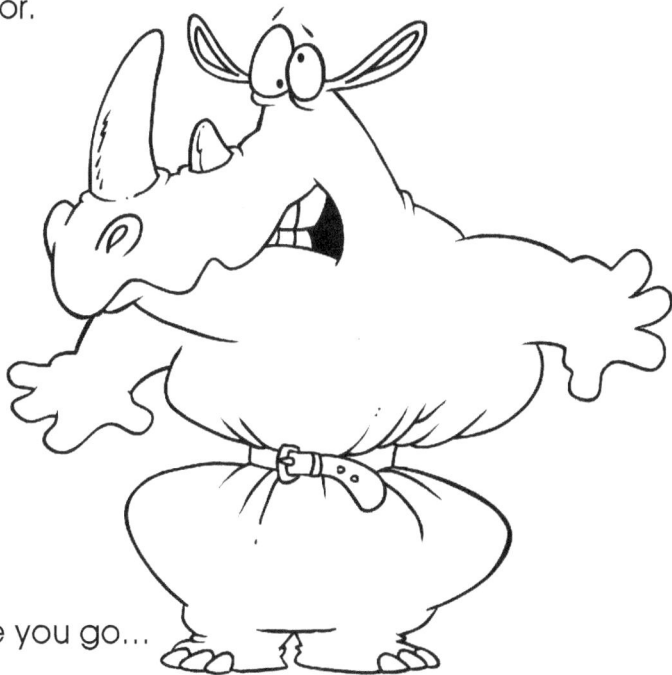

So here you go...

• **Eat as if you're already your ideal weight**. For example, let's say I'm 175 and I want to get down to 155. I'd keep a mental picture of me weighing 155 and as I go through my day, that picture would help me trim back on how much I eat. Therefore I might graze a little less, be more conscious of not overstuffing myself, or go out and take a spontaneous walk.

• **Serve yourself slightly smaller portions.** No need to go measuring anything; in your gut you know how much you usually put on your plate. Just get in the habit of making a conscious effort to put *slightly* less on your plate. If you're still hungry, go back for more.

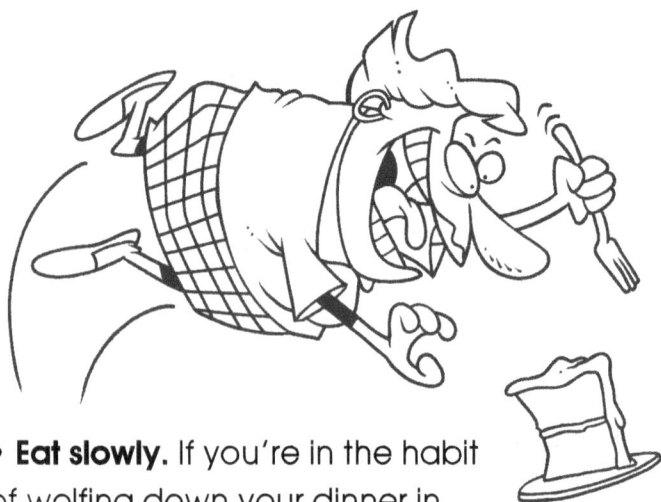

• **Eat slowly.** If you're in the habit of wolfing down your dinner in 15 minutes, (which I usually do) you need to do it in 20 minutes instead. Look at the clock and become more aware of how much time it takes you to eat a meal. When you eat slower, you give your brain more time to receive the "full" signal from your stomach and therefore you'll be less apt to eat more than you need to.

• **Leave the last 5%.** If you consume 2,000 calories a day, by getting in the habit of leaving the last 5% of your food on your plate, you'll trim back 100 calories a day.

• **Swap it.** Find substitutes for the high-calorie foods you consume. For example, if you swap 2 oz. of fat-free yogurt for 2 oz. of heavy cream, you'll lower your calories by 170. Two handfuls of oil-roasted mixed nuts have 350 calories while two handfuls of pistachio nuts (with shells) have 159 calories.

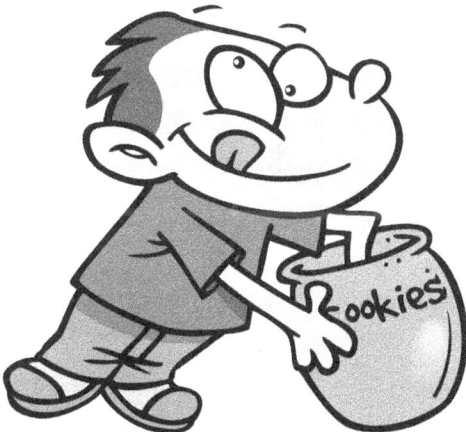

• **Ease up on dessert.** If you like having a few cookies after dinner, have two cookies instead of three. A 1 oz. chocolate chip cookie, for example, is 148 calories. That translates to 15 pounds a year if you did nothing other than cut out one "CCC" a day.

• **Wait a half hour before you snarf down dessert.** Whenever I do, I find that I usually don't want as much dessert as I originally did. This one technique alone makes it effortless (and I mean effortless) to trim back over 100 calories a day.

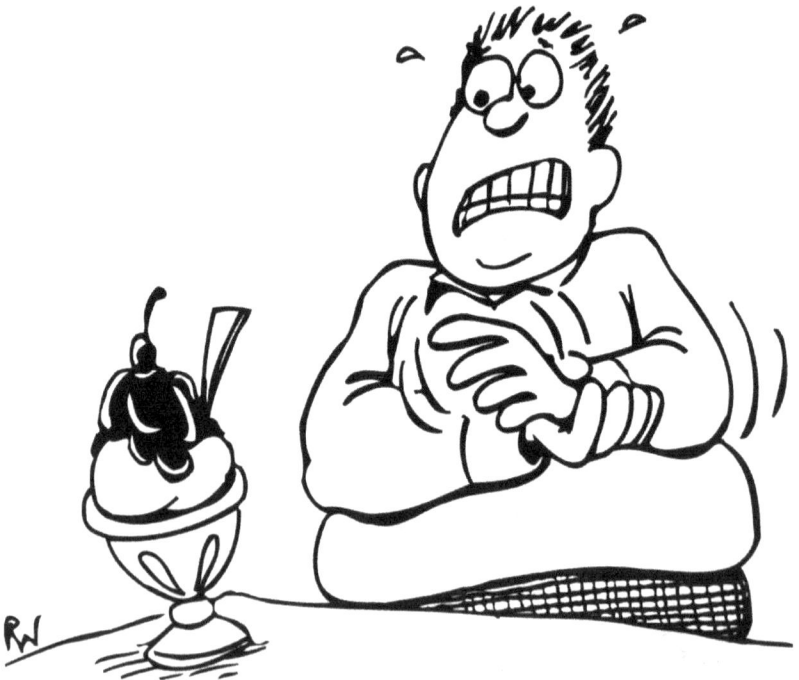

• **Snack on veggies or fruit throughout the day.** Keep carrots or celery handy and munch on them as much as you'd like. In a relatively short period of time, you'll build up a new habit for yourself. If you want a candy bar instead, go ahead and have your candy bar. If you want to stop the veggie-fest, go ahead stop the veggie-fest and then try some other approach. Once again, when you're on *The Turtle Diet*, it's impossible to fall off. If you feel like you're doing something that's really hard, then don't do it. Allow time (i.e. losing weight over the course of weeks or months rather than days) to work for you.

• **Put the veggies (and fruits, too) front and center.** By that I mean place the carrots and celery right at eye level in the refrigerator so the moment you open the door, you can't miss them. Make sure that you take them out of the bag, clean them and slice them so that they're ready to go. Make it a cinch to pop them in your mouth. Recently I was frustrated that my kids weren't eating enough fruits and

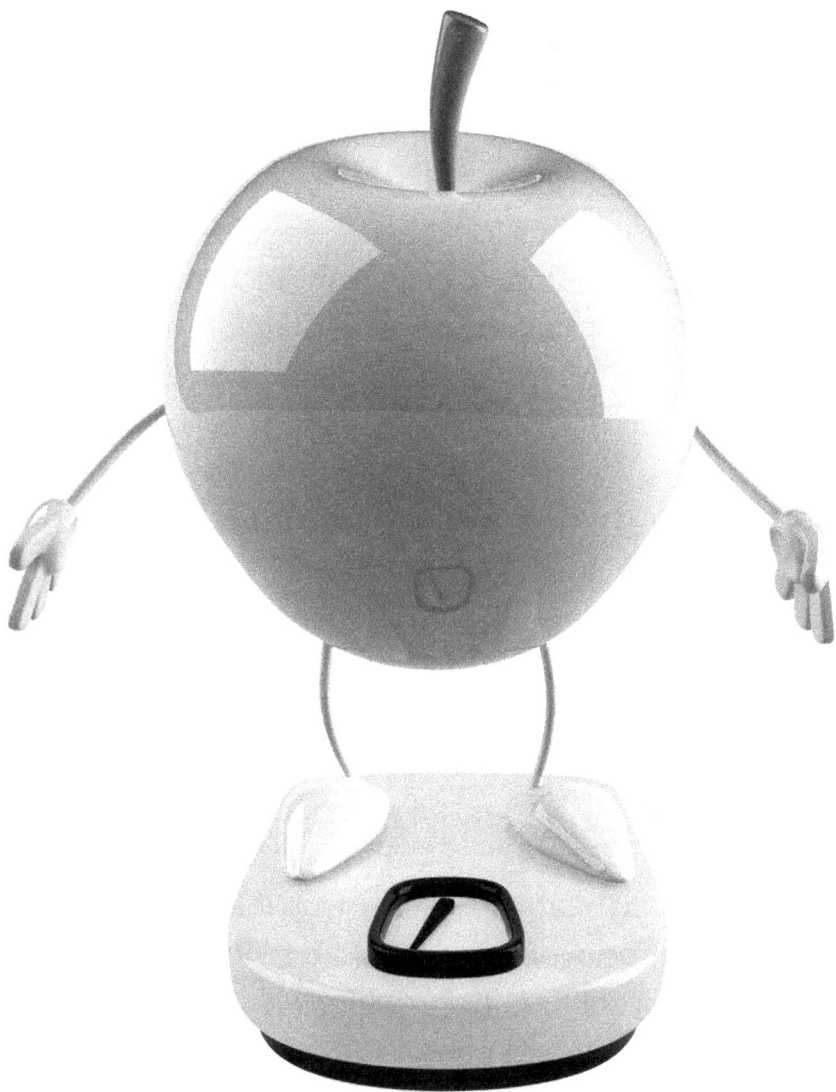

vegetables. We had plenty of healthy food in the refrigerator, but it just wasn't being eaten because it wasn't visible. It was hidden in the fruit and vegetable bin and the kids would never look in there. But as soon as I took it out of the drawer and put it smack on the front of the shelf, it got munched.

• **Try not to eat too late in the evening.** Allow two or three hours between the time you have your last bite and when you go to bed. This allows your body time to better digest and burn off the calories you consumed. It'll also help you sleep better.

• **Ask yourself:** Is the choice I'm about to make going to get me closer to where I want to go? So as you reach for that big second helping or before you gobble up that fourth cookie, get in the habit of asking yourself that question. The answer you come up with will help guide you.

I could list a dozen more ideas (low fat, high fiber, less sugar, more whole grains, yada, yada) but I'm not going to. I promised at the outset that I wasn't going to drown you in details. This book is about giving you a simple framework. What you need to do is find the one or two new behaviors that will work easily for you and start doing them little by little. The cool thing is that once you see results, you'll be self-motivated to keep up with the new behaviors and maybe even try a couple more behaviors. Success breeds success.

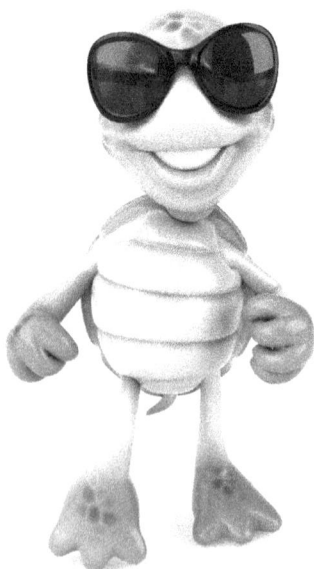

The first law of dietetics seems to be that if it tastes good, it's bad for you.

Isaac Asimov

9. Gulp Gulp

I like soda. Always have. On average, I probably drink about a can and a half a day. That may not sound too bad, but it translates to about 230 calories per day (equivalent to 15 teaspoons of sugar). Oh boy. Theoretically, if I did nothing else but cut out full calorie soda, I'd consume 85,410 less calories every year. And how many pounds does that equal? Well, 85,410 divided by 3,500 (the number of calories in a pound of fat) equals 24 pounds. You got to be kidding! If I did nothing more than make this one adjustment to my diet, I'd lose two pounds a month and

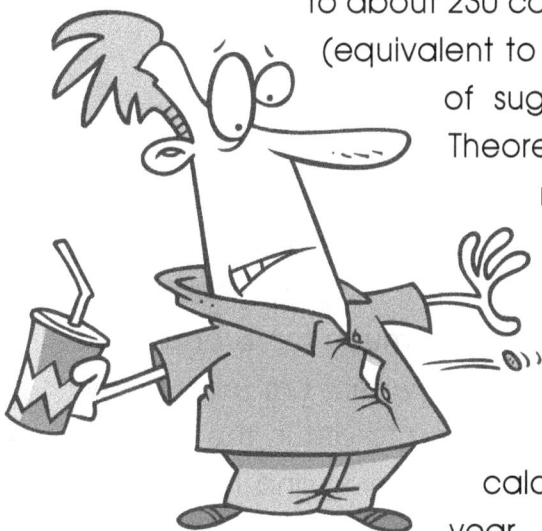

look (and feel) noticeably better.

But what if I couldn't break the soda habit? No problem. I might decide to just drink it every *other* day. This way, I'd still get my fix *and* lose weight, too. When you put time into the equation, all those calories add up.

Here are a few suggestions that will help you when it comes to beverages:

• First and foremost, drink more water. I've never been much of a water drinker. I usually drink it only when I'm thirsty, but since being on *The Turtle Diet*, I'm much more conscious of drinking it even when I'm not thirsty. Lately I've been trying to get in the habit of drinking 12 oz. in the morning and 12 oz. in the afternoon.

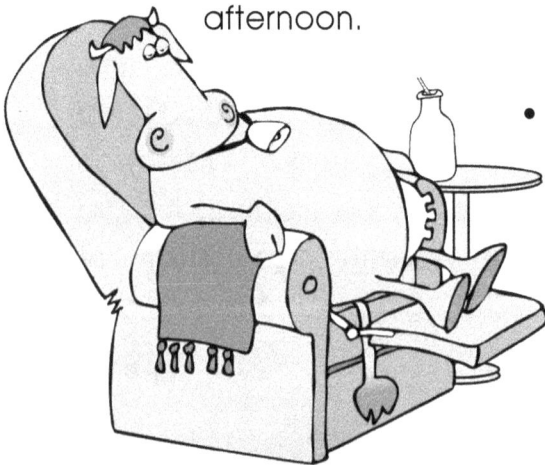

• Switch from regular milk to 2% milk. If you already

drink 2%, go down to 1%. Or go from 1% to skim milk. Each step downward cuts the calories by about 20 percent. An 8 oz. glass of whole milk has 150 calories, while and 8 oz. glass of skim milk has 85 calories. Once you train your taste buds to enjoy skim milk, you could lose a pound every two months from this alone.

• Cut back on the alcohol. If you're a wine drinker, order wine by the glass, not the bottle. When you do it this way, you'll be more aware of how much alcohol (calories) you're drinking.

• Designer coffees pack in lots of calories due to the whole milk, whipped cream, sugar, and syrups. An 8 oz. Starbucks' Caramel Brulee Frappuccino Blended Coffee for example, has 150 calories vs. a

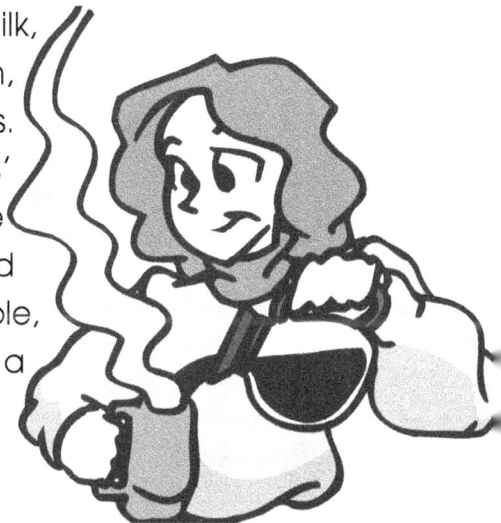

regular 8 oz. Dunkin Donuts coffee with a little milk and sugar, which has about 65 calories.

Here's a short list of some other popular beverages. Which one of these can you trim back? (And let me remind you that 100 calories a day equates to 10 pounds a year.)

- Beer (12 oz.): 146 calories

- Chardonnay (4 oz.): 90 calories

- Whole milk (8 oz.): 150 calories

- Reindeer Milk (8 oz.): 580 calories
  (Just checking to see if you're paying attention.)

- Orange juice (1 cup): 100 calories

- Coca-Cola (12 oz can): 155 calories

- Thick shake (10 oz.): 356 calories

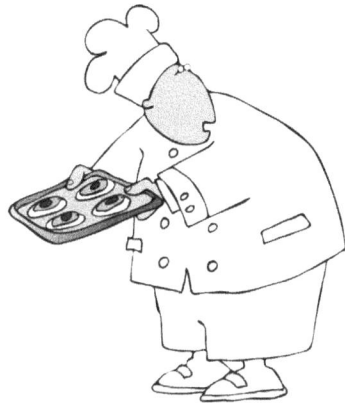

My doctor told me to stop having intimate dinners for four; unless there are three more people there.

Orson Wells

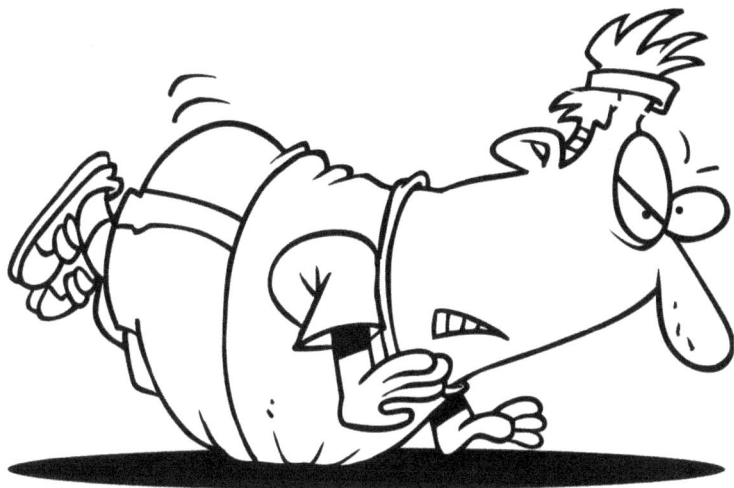

10. Giddyap

The previous two chapters focused on trimming back the amount of calories you consume. By being a little more aware about what you eat and drink and trimming back just a bit, you should be able to hit your goal without too much effort. The other option you have instead of (or in addition to) cutting down on your calories, is to burn off more calories through exercise. For those that don't want to change their eating habits one iota, here's your other option.

Personally, I've never been an exercise nut. While I like to hike, bike ride and swim, I've found that I've never been very good at sustaining a regular exercise regimen. One week I'm all gung-ho and the next week I'm a slug. When you're on *The Turtle Diet*, you don't have to have an intense workout schedule. However, what you do have to do is to make a more conscious effort of doing some little things that help burn calories and, over time, will amount to weight loss.

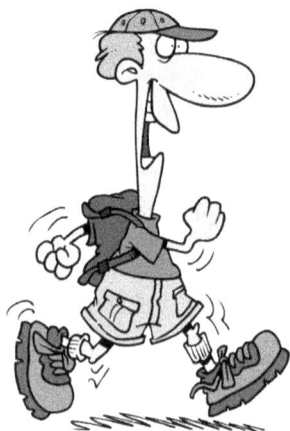

What I'm not going to do is recommend that you work out 5 times a week. While that's an admirable goal, it's totally unrealistic for people who haven't been doing much up to this point.

What most Americans need are some

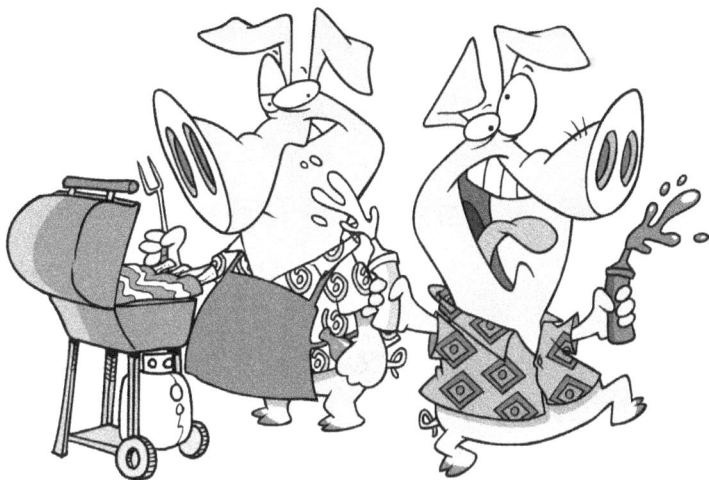

commonsense ideas that are easy to do, can be woven into their day, and don't demand a lifestyle overhaul. In fact, most of the things you see in the list below don't even require that you change into workout clothes.

Let's look at the math once again: If you burn 100 calories more per day than you currently do, you will lose 10 lbs. per year. (This assumes that your weight was stable when you started). If you combine that extra calorie burn with a 100 calorie per day reduction in the amount of calories you consume, you will be down 200 calories every day. That means you'll be 20 pounds lighter this time next year.

Bear in mind that *The Turtle Diet* is not about keeping track of the calories you burn each and every day. That's way too much trouble. Rather, it's about being more conscious of how much you currently exercise (or don't exercise) and then doing a *little* more than you're currently doing.

The list below is based on a 150 lb person doing the activity for 20 minutes. Lighter people will burn fewer calories and heavier people will burn more.

- Basketball: 165 calories
- Bicycling (10 mph): 120 calories
- Housecleaning: 81 calories
- Jogging (5 mph): 200 calories
- Swimming: 138 calories
- Walking casually (3 mph): 45 calories
- Walking briskly (4 mph): 115 calories
- Walking up one flight of stairs: 10 calories
- Yard work: 100 calories

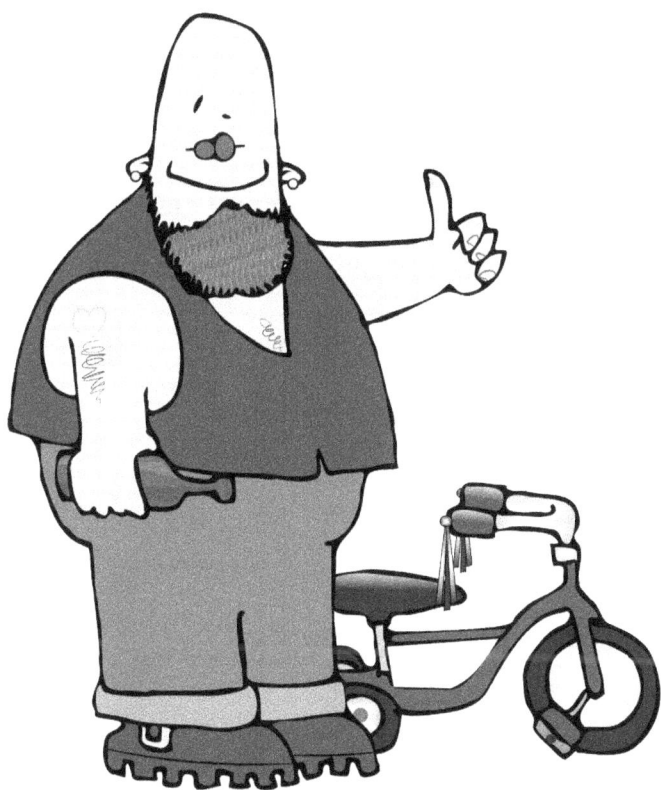

The Centers for Disease Control says that if you spend 10 minutes a day walking up and down stairs, that's all it takes to help you shed as much as 10 pounds a year. Alternatively, you could lose 10 pounds per year if you take a brisk 15 minute (one-mile) walk everyday.

Here are a few online resources where you can find detailed lists of calories burned for a variety of activities:

- www.coolnurse.com/calories.htm
- www.nutristrategy.com/activitylist4.htm
- www.mayoclinic.com/health/exercise/ SM00109

I went to a restaurant that serves breakfast at any time. So I ordered French Toast during the Renaissance.

Stephen Wright

To sum it all up...

Okay, let's see if you were paying attention. Rather than having me sum up the book, how about if you sum it up? Just fill in the blanks below and you'll have the core of *The Turtle Diet*.

1. *The Turtle Diet* is the _____way to lose weight.

2. If you want to lose 10 pounds in one year, you'll have to consume _____ fewer calories per day. In other words: ___ = 10.

3. If you want to lose weight fast, then *The Turtle Diet* is _____.

4. On The *Turtle* Diet, _____ is your best friend.

5. No pain, no _____.

6. If you currently eat four Oreos everyday and cut it back to two Oreos everyday, by the end of one year you will have lost _____ pounds.

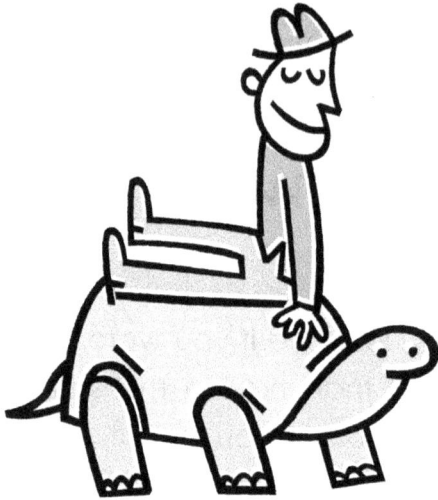

7. It's _____ to fall off *The Turtle Diet*.

8. _____ is the key to your success on *The Turtle Diet*.

9. The essence of *The Turtle Diet* is to make very _____ changes over a _____ period of time.

10. It's important to chart your _____.

You'll find the answers to the above questions on the following pages: *1 - cover, 2 - p.2, 3 - foreword, 4 - p.11, 5 - p.17, 6 - p.5, 7 - p.21, 8 - p.11, 9 - p.12, 10 - p.35.*

The Turtle Diet
is available online.

Health food may be good for the conscience, but Oreos taste a hell of a lot better.

Robert Redford

About the Author
(Kevin Carroll: A life in bullet points)

- The third of seven kids from an Irish Catholic family.

- Grew up just outside New York City.

- Worked in advertising for 17 years.

- Once tried stand-up comedy. (His career was described as "short and dubious.")

- In 1996 got out of advertising (on account of good behavior) and started his own corporate training and consulting business. His motto is: Think Creatively. Communicate Persuasively.

- Most memorable assignment:: teaching conflict resolution at the US Postal Service. (Seriously.)

- Clients have included: Microsoft, Chubb, Wrigley, Pitney Bowes, Unilever, IBM, Fast Company, Gannett, Sikorsky and Staples.

- Written three books: Make Your Point!, Think Outside Your Blocks, and What's Your Hook?

- In 2008, created a family board game (with the help of his daughter and a friend of his) and sold it to a game company. The game's called Pickles to Penguins.

- Married, two kids, one dog, and lives in Connecticut.

Check out Kevin Carroll's
other books online:

_____

Make Your Point!

Think Outside Your Blocks

What's Your Hook?

www.kevincarroll.com

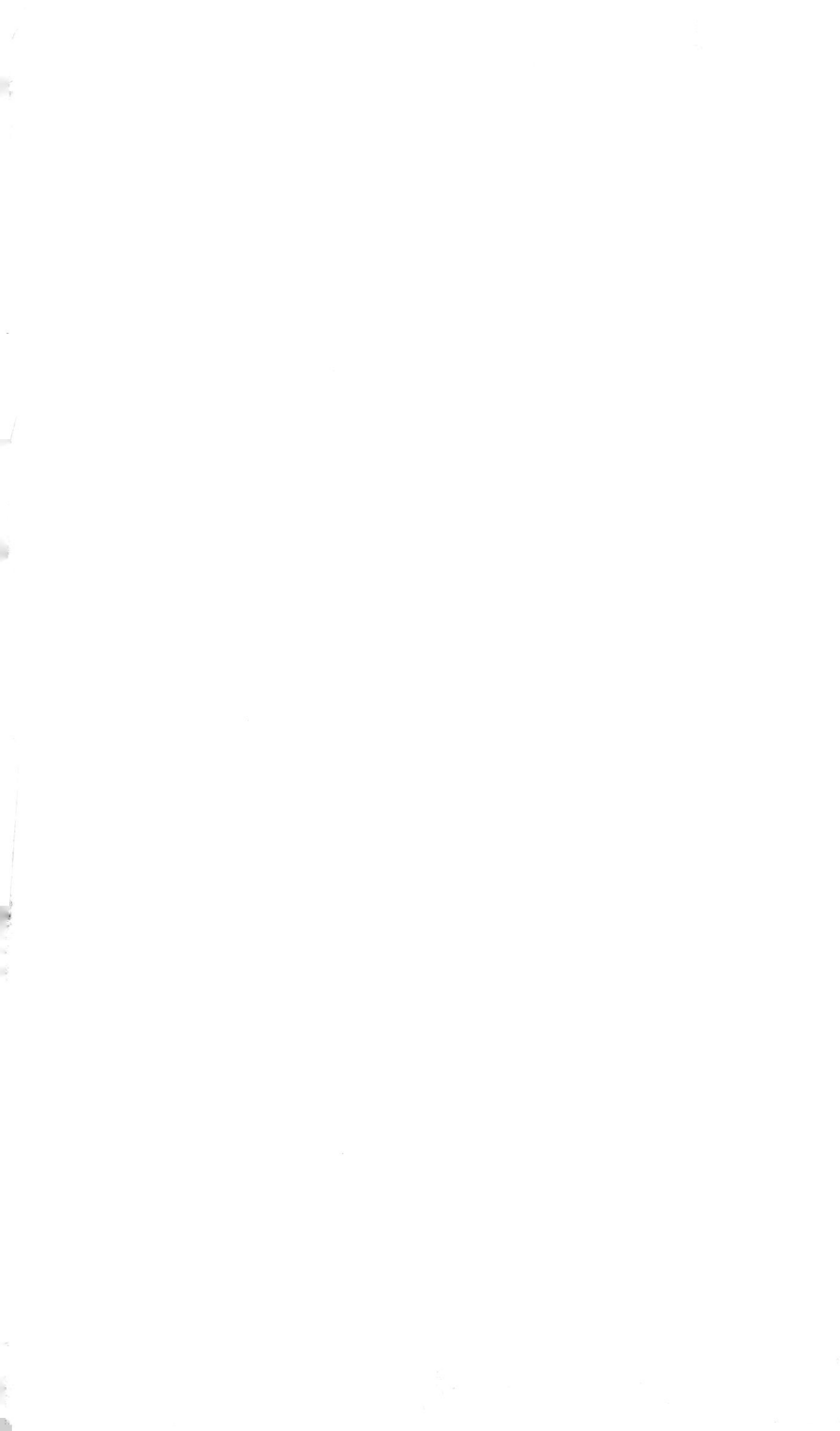

* 9 7 8 0 9 8 1 9 6 0 8 2 1 *